I0479499

Growing Healthy Kids:

A Guide to Prevention and Management of Child Obesity.

Copyright

Table of Content

Introduction

Childhood obesity is a growing concern in today's society. With the rise of processed foods and sedentary lifestyles, children are at a higher risk of developing health problems such as diabetes, heart disease, and high blood pressure. However, there are steps parents and caregivers can take to prevent and manage childhood obesity. This book will serve as a guide to promoting healthy habits for children, including healthy eating, regular exercise, and proper sleep.

It offers evidence-based strategies for preventing and managing obesity in children of all ages, as well as practical advice on nutrition, physical activity, and lifestyle. It also offers detailed information on recognizing and addressing common challenges associated with childhood obesity, including mental health issues and social stigma. With this book, parents and caregivers will be better equipped to help children lead healthier lives.

Chapter 1:

Understanding Child Obesity

This chapter will outline what childhood obesity is and why it is a problem. It will explore the causes of child obesity, including genetics, environment, and lifestyle factors. The chapter will also discuss the health risks associated with childhood obesity and how it can impact a child's physical and mental health.

What is childhood obesity and why it is a problem?

Child obesity is a condition where a child has an excess amount of body fat that can lead to negative health outcomes. It is not just a cosmetic concern, but a serious medical condition that can have long-term health effects. Obesity in children is determined by a Body Mass Index (BMI) calculation that takes into account a child's height and weight. A BMI above 85% for children of the same age and sex is considered overweight, and a BMI above 95% is considered obese.

Child obesity is a problem because it can lead to a range of health issues that can have a significant impact on a child's life. Obese children are at risk of developing health problems such as type 2 diabetes, high blood pressure, and high cholesterol, all of which can increase their risk of heart disease and stroke later in life. Obese children are also at risk of developing joint problems, sleep apnea, and liver disease. They may also experience social and emotional difficulties due to bullying, low self-esteem, and depression.

Moreover, child obesity can also have economic and social implications. Obese children may require more medical care and are more likely to miss school due to illness. They may also experience discrimination and stigmatization, which can lead to social isolation and other negative outcomes.

Child obesity is a significant problem that can have long-term health, social, and economic consequences. It is crucial to recognize the problem and take necessary steps to prevent and manage it to ensure that our children grow up healthy and happy.

The causes of childhood obesity

Child obesity is a complex condition with multiple causes, including genetics, environment, and lifestyle factors. The following factors can contribute to the development of child obesity:

Genetics:

Research has shown that genetics play a role in child obesity. Children with a family history of obesity are more likely to develop obesity themselves. However, genetics alone cannot explain the increase in child obesity rates in recent years.

Environment:

The environment in which a child grows up can have a significant impact on their weight. Children who live in neighborhoods with limited access to healthy food options, such as fresh fruits and vegetables, are more likely to consume high-calorie, high-fat foods. Additionally, children who live in neighborhoods without safe places to exercise may not get enough physical activity.

Lifestyle factors:
Lifestyle factors such as diet and physical activity play a significant role in the development of child

obesity. Children who consume high-calorie, high-fat foods and sugary drinks are more likely to become overweight or obese. Similarly, children who do not get enough physical activity are at risk of gaining excess weight.

Other factors:
Other factors that can contribute to child obesity include socioeconomic status, parenting practices,

and cultural factors. Children from low-income families may be more likely to become obese due to limited access to healthy food options and safe places to exercise. Parenting practices, such as using food as a reward or comfort, can also contribute to weight gain. Cultural factors, such as the prevalence of fast food restaurants and sedentary lifestyles, can also contribute to child obesity.

Health risks associated with childhood obesity and how it can impact a child's physical and mental health. Childhood obesity can have a range of negative health consequences that can impact a child's physical and mental health. The health risks associated with childhood obesity include:

Type 2 diabetes: Obese children are at risk of developing type 2 diabetes, a condition where the body does not produce or use insulin properly. This can lead to high blood sugar levels, which can cause damage to organs and tissues over time.

High blood pressure: Obese children are at risk of developing high blood pressure, which can increase the risk of heart disease and stroke later in life.

High cholesterol: Obese children may have high levels of cholesterol, which can increase the risk of heart disease.

Asthma: Obese children are at risk of developing asthma, a condition that causes difficulty breathing.

Sleep apnea: Obese children may develop sleep apnea, a condition where breathing is disrupted during sleep.

Joint problems: Obese children are at risk of developing joint problems, such as arthritis, due to the excess weight on their joints.

Mental health problems: Obese children may experience social and emotional difficulties, such as low self-esteem, depression, and anxiety, due to bullying and stigmatization.

In addition to these health risks, childhood obesity can also impact a child's quality of life. Obese children may have difficulty participating in physical activities, which can impact their social development and academic performance. They may also experience discrimination and stigmatization, which can lead to social isolation and other negative outcomes.

Childhood obesity is a serious medical condition that can have long-term health consequences and impact a child's physical and mental health. It is crucial to recognize the problem and take necessary steps to prevent and manage it to ensure that our children grow up healthy and happy.

In conclusion, child obesity is a complex condition with multiple causes, including genetics, environment, and lifestyle factors. Understanding these factors is crucial in preventing and managing child obesity. By creating a supportive environment and promoting healthy habits, we can help our children lead healthy and happy lives.

The Role of Nutrition in Child Obesity

Nutrition plays a significant role in the development of childhood obesity. Poor nutrition can contribute to weight gain and increased risk of obesity in children. Consuming too many calories, particularly from unhealthy sources such as sugary drinks and processed foods, should be discouraged.

Caloric Intake:

Children who consume more calories than they burn off through physical activity and daily functioning are at risk for weight gain and obesity. A diet high in high-calorie, high-fat, and high-sugar foods can contribute to the development of obesity.

Portion Control:

Portion control is essential in managing childhood obesity. Parents should encourage their children to eat appropriate portion sizes and avoid overeating. This can be achieved by serving smaller portions, using smaller plates, and avoiding second helpings.

Healthy Foods:

Parents and caregivers should provide a healthy

and balanced diet for their children. This includes a variety of fruits, vegetables, whole grains, lean protein sources, and low-fat dairy products. It is important to limit the intake of sugary drinks, processed foods, and snacks high in fat and sugar.

Nutritional Education:
Education about the
importance of nutrition is
critical for helping children
to maintain a healthy
weight. Teaching children
about healthy eating can
help to prevent childhood
obesity. Parents and
caregivers can teach
children about healthy food
choices, the importance of
balanced meals, and how to
read food labels. This can
help children make

informed choices about their food intake.

Nutrient-Rich Foods to Improve Health

Fruits and Vegetables – Fruits and vegetables are chock-full of essential vitamins and minerals, as well as dietary fiber, which can help keep kids feeling full for longer and provide lasting energy. Offer a variety of colorful fruits and vegetables to ensure your child is getting a wide range of nutrients.

Whole Grains – Whole grains, such as oats, quinoa, and brown rice, are a great source of complex carbohydrates that can provide your child with lasting energy. They also provide essential vitamins, minerals, and dietary fiber.

Lean Proteins – Lean proteins, such as chicken, fish, eggs, and beans, are a great source of essential amino acids that are necessary for growth and development.

Dairy – Dairy products, such as milk, yogurt, and cheese, are an excellent source of calcium and vitamin D, which are both important for bone health.

Nuts and Seeds – Nuts and seeds are a great source of healthy fats, as well as essential vitamins and minerals. They can be a great snack option for kids and adults alike.

Healthy Fats – Healthy fats, such as those found in avocados, olive oil, and nut kinds of butter, are a great way to provide your child with essential fatty acids that are necessary for proper growth and development.

Challenges of Ensuring Nutritional Needs Are Met

Ensuring that a balanced diet is consumed: A balanced diet is essential for maintaining good health, however, it can be difficult to ensure that all essential nutrients are consumed.

Meeting dietary restrictions and allergies: Many individuals have dietary restrictions or allergies that must be taken into account when planning meals, so making sure all dietary needs are met can be a challenge.

Sticking to a budget: Nutritious foods can often be more expensive, making it difficult to stay within a budget and still meet nutritional needs.

Planning meals and snacks: Planning meals and snacks that are nutritious and provide enough energy for the day can be a challenge.

Finding nutritious food options away from home: When eating away from home, it can be difficult to find nutritious food options.

Making out time for cooking: With busy lifestyles, it can be difficult to make time to cook nutritious meals.

Encouraging children to make healthy choices: It can be challenging to encourage children to make healthy choices when it comes to food.

Dealing with picky eaters: Picky eaters can make it difficult to ensure that nutritional needs are met.

Avoiding unhealthy snacks and processed foods: It can be difficult to avoid unhealthy snacks and processed foods that are high in calories and low in nutritional value.

Making healthy eating enjoyable: Eating healthy can be boring and unappealing, making it difficult to make healthy eating an enjoyable experience.

Strategies Parents can adopt for Promoting Healthy Eating and Physical Activities in combating childhood obesity

1. **Serve healthy meals and snacks regularly**: Offer a variety of nutritious foods at meal and snack times to ensure your child is getting the vitamins, minerals, and other nutrients they need.

2. **Make physical activity a priority**: Encourage your child to be active every day by setting aside time for physical activity.

3. **Lead by example**: Set a good example for your child by leading a healthy lifestyle yourself and maintaining a healthy diet.

4. **Limit screen time**:

Limit the amount of time your child spends in front of the TV, computer, tablet, or phone each day.

5. **Educate your child about nutrition**: Help your child understand the importance of making healthy food choices and staying active.

6. **Involve your child in food preparation**: Involve your child in the food preparation process to help make healthy eating fun.

7. **Choose healthy snacks**: Offer your child healthy snacks such as fruits, vegetables, and nuts instead of sugary snacks and drinks.

8. **Make meals a family affair**: Make mealtime a family affair by eating

together as much as possible.

9. Find ways to make physical activity fun: Encourage your child to be active by finding fun ways to be physically active such as playing tag, going for a walk, or playing a game of catch.

10. Praise your child for healthy eating and physical activity: Make sure to praise and encourage your child when they make healthy food choices and stay active.

In conclusion, nutrition plays a significant role in the development of childhood obesity. By encouraging appropriate caloric intake, portion control, healthy food choices, and nutritional education, parents and caregivers can help their children develop healthy eating habits that will last a lifetime.

Strategies for Encouraging Physical Activity

Set Goals and Track Progress: Setting specific goals and tracking your progress can help you stay motivated and on track to reach your fitness goals.

Creating a plan and tracking your progress can help you stay focused and motivated to reach your desired outcome.

Exercise with a Friend or Group: Exercising with

a friend or group can make physical activity more enjoyable and help you stay motivated. Working out with someone else can also provide you with accountability and a support system that can help keep you motivated and on track.

Try Something New: If you're feeling bored with your current routine, try something new! You may find that a new activity or exercise program can help reignite your motivation and make physical activity more enjoyable.

Create Rewards:

Creating rewards for yourself can help you stay motivated and encourage you to keep up with your physical activity routine. These rewards can include anything from a piece of chocolate to a new piece of exercise equipment.

Change Up Your Routine: It's easy to get into a rut when it comes to physical activity. Try switching up your routine to keep things fresh and exciting. You may find that adding variety to your routine makes it easier to stay motivated and engaged.

Set Realistic Expectations: Setting realistic expectations for yourself can help you stay focused and motivated to reach your goals. Having a realistic plan and timeline for achieving your desired outcomes can help you stay on track and avoid disappointment.

Make Exercise Fun: Exercise doesn't have to be boring. Find activities that you enjoy and make them part of your routine. You may find that making physical activity fun and exciting can help you stay motivated and engaged.

Break it Up: If you're having trouble finding the time to fit physical activity into your daily routine, try breaking it up into smaller chunks. You may find that taking 10-15 minutes out of each day for physical activity can help you stay on track and keep your motivation levels high.

Chapter 2:

Building Healthy Habits

This chapter will focus on building healthy habits through healthy eating, regular exercise, and proper sleep. It will provide practical tips for parents and caregivers to ensure that children are getting the nutrients they need from a balanced diet, as well as engaging in physical activity on a regular basis. The chapter will also emphasize the importance of proper sleep and how it can impact a child's overall health.

Building healthy habits through healthy eating, regular exercise, and proper sleep.

Building healthy habits is essential for overall health and well-being. Healthy habits such as healthy eating, regular exercise, and proper sleep can help prevent chronic diseases and maintain a healthy weight.

Healthy Eating:

Healthy eating involves consuming a balanced diet that includes a variety of foods from all food groups. Children should consume plenty of fruits, vegetables, whole grains, lean protein, and low-fat dairy products. Parents can encourage healthy eating by involving children in meal planning and preparation, offering healthy snacks, and limiting sugary and high-calorie foods and drinks.

Regular Exercise: Regular exercise is crucial for building strong muscles and bones, maintaining a healthy weight, and reducing the risk of chronic diseases. Children should aim for at least 60 minutes of physical activity every day, which can include activities such as running, swimming, biking, and playing outdoors. Parents can encourage regular exercise by providing opportunities for physical activity, such as joining sports teams or going for family walks.

Proper Sleep:

Proper sleep is essential for physical and mental health. Children should aim for 9-12 hours of sleep each night, depending on their age. Parents can promote proper sleep by establishing a regular bedtime routine, limiting screen time before bed, and creating a quiet and comfortable sleep environment.

Building healthy habits through healthy eating, regular exercise, and proper sleep is crucial for maintaining good health and preventing chronic diseases. By promoting healthy habits from a young age, we can help our children lead healthy and happy lives.

Practical tips for parents and caregivers to ensure

that children are getting the nutrients they need from a balanced diet, as well as engaging in physical activity on a regular basis.

Here are some practical tips for parents and caregivers to ensure that children are getting the nutrients they need from a balanced diet and engaging in physical activity on a regular basis:

Plan meals and snacks ahead of time: Plan meals and snacks ahead of time to ensure that children are getting a variety of nutrient-dense foods. Include a variety of fruits, vegetables, whole grains, lean proteins, and low-fat dairy products in their diet.

Get children involved in meal planning and preparation: Involve children in meal planning and preparation to encourage healthy eating habits. Let them choose healthy foods they enjoy, and allow them to help with meal prep and cooking.

Offer healthy snacks: Offer healthy snacks, such as fruits, vegetables, and whole-grain crackers, instead of sugary snacks and drinks.

Encourage physical activity: Encourage physical activity by providing opportunities for exercise, such as going for family walks, bike rides, or playing outdoors. Limit screen time and encourage children to engage in physical activity for at least 60 minutes a day.

Be a role model: Be a role model for healthy eating and physical activity. Children are more likely to adopt healthy habits when they see their parents and caregivers modeling healthy behaviors.

Make it fun: Make healthy eating and physical activity fun for children. Involve them in activities that they enjoy, such as dancing, swimming, or playing games.

By planning meals and snacks ahead of time, involving children in meal planning and preparation, offering healthy snacks, encouraging physical activity, being a role model, and making it fun, parents and caregivers can ensure that children are getting the nutrients they need from a balanced diet and engaging in physical activity on a regular basis.

Chapter 3:

Creating a Supportive Environment

This chapter will address the importance of creating a supportive environment for children to foster healthy habits. It will discuss how parents and caregivers can create a positive and supportive atmosphere to promote healthy eating and regular exercise. The chapter will also touch on the role of schools and communities in promoting healthy habits for children.

The importance of creating a supportive environment for children to foster healthy habits.

Creating a supportive environment for children is crucial for fostering healthy habits. A supportive environment can include factors such as access to healthy foods and safe places to play, parental support, and positive social norms.

Access to Healthy Foods:

Access to healthy foods is essential for maintaining a healthy diet. Parents and caregivers can create a supportive environment by providing a variety of healthy foods and limiting access to unhealthy foods and drinks. They can also involve children in meal planning and preparation to encourage healthy eating habits.

Safe Places to Play:

Safe places to play are crucial for physical activity. Parents and caregivers can create a supportive environment by providing opportunities for physical activity, such as going for family walks, bike rides, or playing outdoors. They can also limit screen time and encourage children to engage in physical activity for at least 60 minutes a day.

Parental Support:
Parental support is vital for creating a supportive environment. Parents and caregivers can support healthy habits by being positive role models, offering encouragement and praise, and providing opportunities for children to learn and practice healthy habits.

Limit Sedentary Activities: Encourage children to limit their time spent in sedentary activities such as watching TV, playing video games, or using the internet. This could include placing limits on the amount of time spent on these activities, offering alternative activities such as outdoor play or providing incentives for children to engage in physical activities.

Positive Social Norms: Positive social norms can also contribute to a supportive environment.

When healthy eating and physical activity are valued and encouraged in the community, children are more likely to adopt these habits.

In conclusion, creating a supportive environment for children is critical for fostering healthy habits. By providing access to healthy foods and safe places to play, offering parental support, and promoting positive social norms, parents and caregivers can help children develop healthy habits that will last a lifetime.

The role of schools and communities in promoting healthy habits for children. Schools and communities can play a vital role in promoting healthy habits for children which may include:

Creating a school-wide Initiative that Promotes healthy eating and physical activity

- Educating students on nutrition and the importance of exercise

- Providing healthy snacks and meals in the cafeteria
- Encouraging teachers to incorporate physical activity into their lesson plans, and offering extracurricular activities that involve physical activity.

Here are some ways in which schools and communities can contribute:

Growing Healthy Kids

Health Education:
Schools can teach children the value of eating a well-balanced and nutritious diet. This could include nutrition-related classroom lessons, introducing them to food labels so they can make informed decisions about what they eat, and encouraging them to try new healthy foods. Physical activities and good sleeping habits should also be included. Health education

can teach children the value of healthy habits and how to develop them.

Access to Healthy Foods:

Schools can provide access to healthy foods by offering nutritious school meals, promoting healthy snacks, and limiting access to unhealthy foods and drinks.

Promote Physical Activity:

Encourage children to be active by providing them with opportunities to engage in physical activities. This could include offering after-school sports clubs, organizing school-wide physical activity events, or introducing physical activity into the school curriculum.

Safe Places to Play:

Communities can provide safe places to play, such as parks and playgrounds, to encourage physical activity.

Involve Parents:

Invite parents to get involved in promoting healthy eating and physical activity in their children by providing them with resources and education on the topic. This could include offering nutrition classes, introducing healthy meal planning and cooking tips, or providing them with access to healthy snacks and meals.

Lead by Example:
As a role model, it is critical to set a good example and exhibit healthy behaviors. Making healthy food choices, engaging in physical activities, and limiting sedentary activities are all examples of this. You can set a good example for the children in your care by demonstrating the importance of developing and maintaining healthy habits.

Monitor Progress:

Keep track of your student's progress toward developing healthy habits and intervene as needed. This could include weighing in on a regular basis, assessing physical activity levels, and assessing dietary intake. It is also critical to monitor and assess any behavioral changes that may be related to the development of healthy habits.

Seek Professional Help: Consult a specialist if you are worried about a student's health. This can entail speaking with a nutritionist, dietician, or medical professional. Also, it's critical to offer families who might require assistance in managing their child's health resources and support.

Collaboration:

Schools and communities can collaborate to promote healthy habits for children. For example, schools can partner with community organizations to offer nutrition and physical activity programs, and communities can support schools by promoting healthy habits and providing resources.

Policy Change:

Schools and communities can advocate for policy change to support healthy habits for children. This can include policies to promote healthy school meals, limit access to unhealthy foods and drinks, and provide safe places to play.

Chapter 4:

Managing Child Obesity

This chapter will provide guidance on how to manage child obesity through diet, exercise, and other interventions. It will outline the different treatment options available, including medical interventions and lifestyle changes. The chapter will also address the emotional and psychological impact of childhood obesity and how to support children in a positive and effective way.

Guidance on how to manage child obesity through diet, exercise, and other interventions. Childhood obesity is a serious medical condition that requires careful management. Here is some guidance on how to manage child obesity through diet, exercise, and other interventions:

Healthy Diet:

A healthy diet is essential for managing child obesity. Parents should work with a registered dietitian to develop a healthy meal plan that is tailored to their child's needs. The meal plan should include a variety of nutrient-dense foods, such as fruits, vegetables, whole grains, lean proteins, and low-fat dairy products. Parents should also limit their child's intake of processed and high-calorie foods and drinks, such as sugary drinks, candy, and fast food.

Regular Exercise:

Regular exercise is crucial for managing child obesity. Children should aim for at least 60 minutes of physical activity every day, which can include activities such as running, swimming, biking, and playing outdoors. Parents can encourage regular exercise by providing opportunities for physical activity, such as joining sports teams or going for family walks.

Behavior Modification: Behavior modification techniques can be used to help children adopt healthy habits. Parents can work with a healthcare professional to develop a behavior modification plan that includes setting goals, tracking progress, and rewarding positive behaviors.

Family Support:

Family support is vital for managing child obesity. Parents can provide emotional support and encouragement to their children, help them develop healthy habits, and model healthy behaviors themselves.

Medical Intervention:

In some cases, medical intervention may be necessary to manage child obesity. This can include medication, surgery, or other medical treatments. Parents should work with their healthcare professionals to determine the best course of treatment for their child.

Surgery:

Surgery may be recommended in some cases for children with severe obesity who have not responded to lifestyle changes and other treatment options. Bariatric surgery is a type of surgery that reduces the size of the stomach to limit the amount of food a person can eat.

Managing childhood obesity requires a comprehensive approach that includes lifestyle changes, behavioral therapy, medications, and surgery. Parents should work with a healthcare professional to develop a personalized plan for their child that takes into account their individual needs and circumstances.

The emotional and psychological impact of childhood obesity and how to support children in a positive and effective way.

Childhood obesity can have a significant emotional and psychological impact on children, including low self-esteem, poor body image, and depression. It is important for parents and caregivers to provide emotional support and create a positive and supportive environment for their child.

Encourage Positive Self-Image:

Parents and caregivers should encourage a positive self-image by focusing on their child's strengths and accomplishments, rather than their weight. They can also help their child develop a positive body image by encouraging them to participate in activities that they enjoy and feel good about.

Avoid Stigmatizing Language:

Parents and caregivers should avoid stigmatizing language and negative comments about their child's weight or body size. This can be hurtful and damaging to a child's self-esteem.

Focus on Health, Not Weight:

Parents and caregivers should focus on promoting healthy habits, rather than weight loss. This can include encouraging regular physical activity, providing healthy meals and snacks, and modeling healthy behaviors.

Seek Professional Support:

Parents and caregivers may also want to seek

professional support for their child, such as counseling or support groups. This can provide additional emotional support and help their child develop coping strategies.

Addressing the emotional and psychological impact of childhood obesity requires a supportive and positive environment. By encouraging a positive self-image, avoiding stigmatizing language, focusing on health rather than weight, and seeking professional support, parents and caregivers can support their child in a positive and effective way.

Conclusion

In conclusion, this book offers a comprehensive guide to preventing and managing childhood obesity in children of all ages. It is designed to help parents, educators, and healthcare providers to understand the causes of childhood obesity and the available strategies for prevention and management. With the help of this book, parents can be empowered to take charge of their child's health and put them on the path to a healthier future.

It is important to remember that preventing and managing childhood obesity is a family effort. It takes a village to raise a child, and working together to develop and maintain healthy habits is the best way to ensure the wellbeing of our kids. With this book, readers can learn how to provide a healthy environment for their children and how to promote and maintain a healthy lifestyle.

Thank you for taking the time to read this book and for being an advocate for the health of our children. With the help of this book, we can all work together to create a healthier future for our children.